MACROBIOTIC DIET COOKBOOK

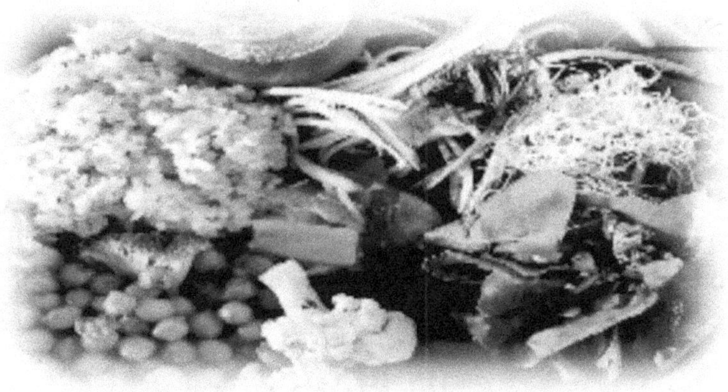

A Beginner's Guide to the 60 Satisfying Recipes to Lose Weight and Gain Lean Muscle for a Balanced Healthy Lifestyle

Dr. Laura Loeffler

Copyright © 2023 by Dr. Laura Loeffler

SCAN TO GAIN ACCESS TO MORE OF MY BOOKS

TABLE OF CONTENTS

INTRODUCTION --5

CHAPITRE 1 ---7

What exactly is the macrobiotic diet?-----------------------7

The Macrobiotic Diet's Scientific Basis--------------------7

The Benefits of the Macrobiotic Diet-----------------------8

How to Apply Macrobiotic Principles in Daily Life------8

Understanding the Different Food Groups ----------------9

Key Meal Composition Principles in the Macrobiotic Diet--9

Important Takeaways ---10

CHAPTER 2---11

NUTRITIOUS RECIPES FOR MACROBIOTICS DIET ---11

Breakfasts to Start Your Day Right--------------------------11

CHAPTER 3---29

Nourishing Lunches and Satisfying Dinners: Delicious and Balanced --29

CHAPTER 4---55

Snacks, Desserts, and Treats for a Balanced Indulgence - 55

CHAPTER 5--**71**

Salads and Smoothies for a Finding Balance and Flavor 71

CHAPTER 6--**81**

14 DAY MEAL PLANS---**81**

Day 1 ---**81**

Day 2 ---**81**

Day 3 ---**81**

Day 4 ---**81**

Day 5 ---**82**

Day 6 ---**82**

Day 7 ---**82**

Day 8 ---**82**

Day 9 ---**83**

Day 10--**83**

Day 11---**83**

Day 12--**83**

Day 13---**84**

Day 14---**84**

CONCLUSION --**85**

14 DAY MEAL PLANNER JOURNAL------------------**88**

INTRODUCTION

It's easy to lose sight of the significance of real, nourishing meals in a world of fast food and processed products. But what if there was a way to eat that not only nourished your body but also aided in the attainment of optimal health and well-being? Enter the macrobiotic diet, a centuries-old dietary philosophy that stresses complete, unadulterated foods and promotes life balance and harmony.

The macrobiotic diet was a lifeline for my aunt, Amelia. Her health began to deteriorate as she approached her late fifties. She was often fatigued, her joints hurt, and she had high blood pressure and type 2 diabetes. She tried a variety of drugs and lifestyle modifications, but nothing worked.

Amelia came upon a book about the macrobiotic diet one day. She became interested in its concepts and began including more fruits, vegetables, and healthy grains in her diet. She saw a significant change within a few months. Her energy levels rose, her joint discomfort lessened, and her blood pressure and blood sugar levels returned to normal.

Amelia's tale is only one of many that demonstrate the macrobiotic diet's transformational effect. This complete cookbook will lead you on your own path to macrobiotic living, equipping you with the knowledge and skills you need to make informed food and health decisions. You'll learn about the science behind the macrobiotic diet, sample a range of tasty and healthy meals, and learn how to use macrobiotic principles in your daily life.

The macrobiotic diet provides something for everyone, whether you want to enhance your general health, manage chronic diseases, or simply consume more healthy foods. Begin this adventure now and see what a difference genuine, wholesome food can make in your life.

Macrobiotic nutrition is based on a comprehensive and balanced approach to eating, with the goal of fostering well-being and harmony within the body, mind, and soul. The macrobiotic diet is one that stresses the underlying relationship between food and health. It is based on ancient Eastern beliefs.

This dietary philosophy is founded on the notion of balance, with the goal of achieving harmony through the eating of natural, whole foods.

Understanding the macrobiotic diet requires adopting a plant-based diet that focuses on locally sourced, seasonal, and organic vegetables. This diet stresses a conscious, purposeful approach to food selection and preparation, with the goal of achieving physiological equilibrium through the interaction of Yin and Yang forces.

It promotes a broad yet simple diet consisting mostly of nutritious grains, fresh vegetables, legumes, and sea vegetables. The idea is to attain balance by eating meals that complement and balance one another, resulting in a sense of vigor and general wellbeing.

CHAPITRE 1

What exactly is the macrobiotic diet?

The macrobiotic diet is a comprehensive nutritional strategy based on ancient Eastern philosophy that emphasizes balance, harmony, and the connection between food and total well-being. Its guiding philosophy is to eat complete, natural foods that promote health and harmony. Macrobiotics is a way of life that includes not just what you eat but also how you eat, prepare, and live.

The Macrobiotic Diet's Scientific Basis

The macrobiotic diet is founded on the notion of balance, which is derived from the concept of Yin and Yang energies. Foods are classified according to their energy qualities, with a focus on creating balance in every meal.

This diet consists mostly of healthy grains, fresh vegetables, legumes, sea vegetables, and the occasional seafood. The idea is to eat meals that complement the body's inherent energy and promote general wellness.

The macrobiotic diet's emphasis on whole foods is scientifically consistent with current nutritional studies supporting the health advantages of whole grains, vegetables, and plant-based diets.

These foods are high in important nutrients, fiber, and antioxidants, all of which contribute to general health and lower the risk of chronic illnesses including heart disease, diabetes, and some cancers.

The Benefits of the Macrobiotic Diet

Adopting a macrobiotic diet may provide various benefits. It aids in weight loss, boosts energy levels, and promotes general well-being. This diet is frequently lauded for its ability to decrease inflammation, improve digestive health, and boost the body's natural healing processes.

Furthermore, because the diet emphasizes complete, unadulterated foods, followers frequently report greater mental clarity and emotional equilibrium.

How to Apply Macrobiotic Principles in Daily Life

Incorporating macrobiotic concepts into daily life entails taking a deliberate approach to food selection, preparation, and consumption. It entails eating whole, locally obtained foods while avoiding processed and refined meals. Steaming, boiling, and baking are preferred cooking techniques over frying or microwaving because they are thought to maintain the food's inherent nutritional characteristics. Mindful eating, dining in a peaceful atmosphere, and chewing food fully are all important parts of this way of life.

Understanding the Different Food Groups

The macrobiotic diet is centered on the following dietary groups:

1. **Grain Whole:** The diet is built on whole grains such as brown rice, barley, millet, and quinoa. Fiber, vitamins, and minerals abound in these grains. veggies: For their broad nutrient content, fresh, locally obtained veggies, particularly leafy greens, root vegetables, and cruciferous vegetables, are vital.

2. **Beans and legumes:** Protein, fiber, and important elements are found in legumes such as lentils, chickpeas, and adzuki beans.

3. **Sea Vegetables:** Sea vegetables such as nori, kombu, and wakame are high in nutrients like iodine and calcium.

4. **Occasional Fish:** For omega-3 fatty acids, some devotees incorporate tiny quantities of fish.

Key Meal Composition Principles in the Macrobiotic Diet

The macrobiotic diet emphasizes finding balance and harmony in each meal. Some fundamental principles are as follows:

1. **Balance Yin and Yang:** To promote harmony, each meal should have a balance of foods with distinct energy qualities.

2. **Local and Seasonal:** Prioritize locally sourced and seasonal meals for freshness and to fulfill the body's demands throughout the year.

3. **Mindful Eating:** Eat in a relaxed setting, chew food completely, and appreciate each bite consciously. Include a variety of healthy foods while keeping meals simple and easy to digest.

4. **Cooking procedures:** To retain food nutrients and natural tastes, use cooking procedures such as steaming, boiling, and baking.

Important Takeaways

The macrobiotic diet takes a comprehensive approach to nutrition and health. Individuals may improve their overall health and vitality by concentrating on complete, natural foods, balanced meal compositions, and mindful eating. Adopting the macrobiotic diet principles benefits not only physical health but also emotional and mental balance, building a stronger connection between food, health, and a happy existence. Finally, the macrobiotic diet promotes a way of life that focuses on nourishing the body, mind, and spirit rather than just eating.

CHAPTER 2

NUTRITIOUS RECIPES FOR MACROBIOTICS DIET

Breakfasts to Start Your Day Right

White Bean Hummus

Ingredients:

- ✓ 2 cups of cooked white beans, washed and rinsedJuice of 1 lemon
- ✓ ¼ cup extra virgin olive oil
- ✓ ¼ cup sesame tahini
- ✓ 2 garlic cloves
- ✓ ¼ tablespoon of sea salt
- ✓ ¼ tablespoon of cumin
- ✓ ¼ tablespoon of paprika

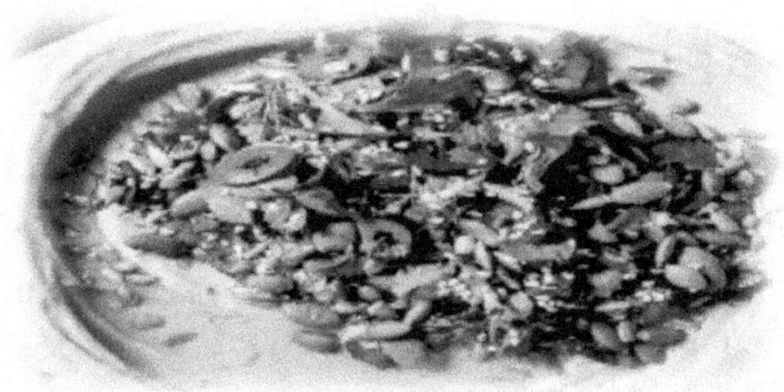

Preparation:

1. Combine all ingredients in a food processor and blend until smooth.

2. Serve with whole grain crackers or vegetables.

Nutritional Value:

This recipe is high in protein, fiber, and healthy fats. White beans are a good source of plant-based protein and fiber, while tahini and olive oil provide healthy fats. Garlic and lemon juice add flavor and antioxidants.

Cooking Time: This recipe takes about 10 minutes to prepare.

Brown Rice Green Bowl

Ingredients:

- ✓ ½ cup cooked brown rice
- ✓ Handful of broccoli florets
- ✓ 2 cups of greens of your choice (baby kale and spinach work well)
- ✓ 2 tsp tamari
- ✓ 1 tsp ume plum vinegar
- ✓ ½ avocado, sliced
- ✓ Dash of sea salt

Preparation:

1. Bring 2-3 tablespoons of water to simmer in a small pot.

2. Add broccoli and cover. Allow to cook for 1-2 minutes until it turns green.

3. Add greens (and a splash more water if the pot is dry), cover and let cook for 1 minute.

4. Add brown rice, tamari, and vinegar to the pot. Stir continuously until everything is warm (about 2 minutes).

5. Transfer to a bowl.

6. Add sliced avocado and a dash of sea salt on top.

Nutritional Value: The recipe has a lot of fiber, vitamins, and minerals. Brown rice is a good source of complex carbohydrates, which provide sustained energy throughout the day. Broccoli and greens are rich in vitamins A and C, as well as calcium and iron. Avocados are high in healthful fats and potassium.

Cooking Time: It takes roughly 10-15 minutes to prepare this dish.

Mediterranean Scrambled Eggs

Ingredients:

✓ 1½ cups halved grape tomatoes

✓ 1 clove garlic, minced

✓ 2 tablespoon of olive oil, divided

✓ 1 (5-oz) pkg baby spinach

✓ 8 large eggs

✓ ½ teaspoon of salt

✓ ½ teaspoon of pepper

✓ ¼ teaspoon of dried oregano

1. Preparation:

1. Cook tomatoes and garlic in 1 tablespoon of hot oil in a large nonstick skillet over medium-high heat 3 to 4 minutes or until tomatoes are tender, stirring occasionally.

2. Add spinach; cook 1 minute or until wilted.

3. Whisk together eggs, salt, pepper, and oregano.

4. Add 1 tablespoon of oil and eggs to skillet; reduce heat to medium.

5. Cook, without stirring, until beginning to set on bottom. Cook, stirring constantly, until thickened and set.

Nutritional Value: This recipe is high in protein, fiber, and vitamins. Eggs are a good source of protein and healthy fats, while spinach and tomatoes provide vitamins and minerals. Olive oil offers antioxidants and healthy fats.

Cooking Time: This recipe takes about 15-20 minutes to prepare.

Vegetable Miso Soup with Mochi Croutons

Ingredients:

✓ 4 cups spring or filtered water

✓ Generous pinch of wakame flakes

✓ 1 cup of daikon radish, cut into half moons

✓ 1 celery stalk, sliced on the diagonal

✓ 2 dried shiitake mushrooms, steeped and sliced overnight (optional)

✓ 3-4 teaspoons organic 3-year barley miso*

✓ 2 green onions, sliced, for garnish

✓ Mochi croutons (see recipe)

Preparation:

1. In a medium soup pot, bring water to a boil with wakame flakes.

2. Add the daikon, celery, shiitake mushrooms, and soaking water for the shiitake mushrooms.

3. Reduce the heat to low and continue to cook for 3-5 minutes, or until the veggies are soft.

4. Purée the miso in ¼ cup broth, then slowly add into the soup until thoroughly combined.

5. Simmer for 2-3 minutes on low heat before serving in bowls with mochi croutons and garnished with green scallions.

Nutritional Value: This meal has a lot of fiber, vitamins, and minerals. Wakame flakes and shiitake mushrooms provide iodine and antioxidants, while daikon and celery add vitamins and minerals. Miso provides probiotics and mochi adds complex carbohydrates.

Cooking Time: This recipe takes about 20-25 minutes to prepare.

Mochi Croutons

Ingredients:

✓ 1 piece of mochi

✓ 1 tsp tamari

✓ 1 tsp sesame oil

Preparation:

1. Preheat oven to 350°F.

2. Cut mochi into small cubes.

3. In a small mixing bowl, combine tamari and sesame oil.

4. Add mochi cubes to the bowl and toss to coat.

5. Place mochi cubes on a baking sheet and bake for 10-15 minutes, until crispy.

Nutritional Value: This recipe is high in complex carbohydrates and provides a good source of energy.

Cooking Time: This recipe takes about 15-20 minutes to prepare.

Tortilla Breakfast Quiche

Ingredients:

✓ 4 whole wheat tortillas

✓ 1 cup cooked quinoa

✓ 1 cup chopped vegetables (e.g. bell peppers, onions, mushrooms)

✓ 4 large eggs

✓ ½ cup unsweetened almond milk

✓ ¼ cup nutritional yeast

✓ ½ teaspoon of sea salt

✓ ¼ teaspoon of black pepper

✓ ¼ teaspoon of dried oregano

✓ ¼ teaspoon of dried basil

✓ ¼ teaspoon of dried thyme

Preparation:

1. Preheat oven to 375°F.

2. Spray a 9-inch pie tin with cooking spray.

3. Place tortillas in the pie dish, overlapping slightly to cover the bottom and sides.

4. Sprinkle cooked quinoa and chopped vegetables over the tortillas.

5. In a medium bowl, whisk together eggs, almond milk, nutritional yeast, sea salt, black pepper, oregano, basil, and thyme.

6. Pour egg mixture over the vegetables.

7. Bake for 25-30 minutes, until the eggs are set and the tortillas are crispy.

8. Allow it cool for a few minutes before cutting it into slices, then serve.

Nutritional Value: This recipe is high in protein, fiber, and vitamins. Eggs are a good source of protein and healthy fats, while vegetables and quinoa provide vitamins and minerals. Nutritional yeast adds a cheesy flavor and provides additional protein and B vitamins.

Cooking Time: This recipe takes about 40-45 minutes to prepare.

Creamy Millet Pudding

Ingredients:

✓ 1 cup millet

✓ 2 cups water

✓ ¼ teaspoon of sea salt

✓ ½ cup unsweetened almond milk

✓ ¼ cup maple syrup

✓ 1 teaspoon of vanilla extract

✓ ¼ teaspoon of cinnamon

Preparation:

1. Rinse millet and drain.

2. Heat a medium-sized pot with the water and salt until they boil.

3. Add millet, reduce heat to low, and simmer for 20-25 minutes, stirring occasionally.

4. Add almond milk, maple syrup, vanilla extract, and cinnamon to the pot. Stir until everything is combined.

5. Serve warm or chilled.

Nutritional Value: This dish is packed in fiber, vitamins, and minerals. Millet is a good source of complex carbohydrates, protein, and fiber. Almond milk provides calcium and vitamin E, while maple syrup adds natural sweetness.

Cooking Time: This recipe takes about 30-35 minutes to prepare.

French Toast Scramble

Ingredients:

✓ 4 slices of whole grain bread

✓ 4 large eggs

✓ ½ cup of unsweetened almond milk

✓ 1 teaspoon of vanilla extract

✓ ½ teaspoon of cinnamon

✓ ¼ teaspoon of nutmeg

✓ 1 tablespoon of coconut oil

✓ 1 tablespoon of maple syrup (optional)

✓ Fresh fruit for serving (optional)

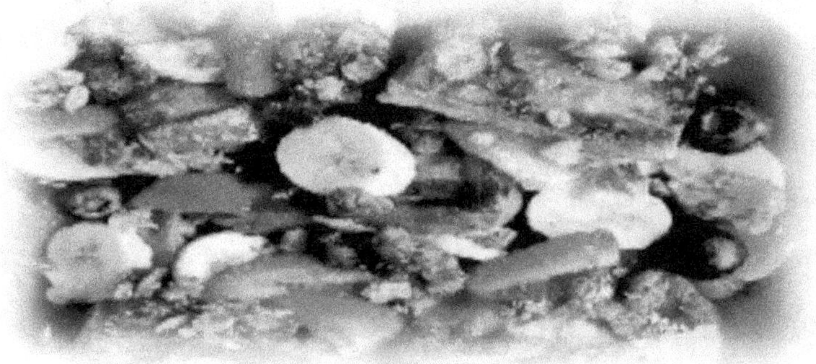

Preparation:

1. In a shallow dish, whisk together eggs, almond milk, vanilla extract, cinnamon, and nutmeg.

2. Coat both sides before dipping each slice of the bread into the egg mixture.

3. In a large nonstick skillet over medium heat, melt the coconut oil.

4. Add the bread slices to the skillet and cook for 2-3 minutes on each side, until golden brown and crispy.

5. Remove the bread from the skillet and cut into small pieces.

6. Return the skillet to the heat and add the leftover egg mixture.

7. Cook the eggs, stirring occasionally, until scrambled and cooked through.

8. Serve the French toast scramble with maple syrup and fresh fruit, if desired.

Nutritional Value: This recipe is high in protein, fiber, and vitamins. Whole grain bread provides complex carbohydrates and fiber, while eggs provide protein and healthy fats. Almond milk adds calcium and vitamin E, while cinnamon and nutmeg provide antioxidants.

Cooking Time: This recipe takes about 15-20 minutes to prepare.

Carrot Cake Overnight Oats

Ingredients:

✓ 1 cup rolled oats

✓ ⅔ cup of unsweetened almond milk

✓ ⅓ cup of grated carrots

✓ 1 tablespoon of chia seeds

✓ 1 tablespoon of maple syrup

✓ ½ teaspoon of cinnamon

✓ ¼ teaspoon of nutmeg

✓ ¼ teaspoon of ginger

✓ ¼ teaspoon of sea salt

✓ Optional toppings: chopped nuts, raisins, shredded coconut

Preparation:

1. In a medium bowl, combine rolled oats, almond milk, grated carrots, chia seeds, maple syrup, cinnamon, nutmeg, ginger, and sea salt.

2. Stir until everything is well combined.

3. Refrigerate the bowl overnight, either in plastic wrap or with a cover.

4. In the morning, stir the oats and add toppings of your choice.

Nutritional Value: This recipe is high in fiber, vitamins, and minerals. Rolled oats are a good source of complex carbohydrates and fiber, while grated carrots provide vitamins and minerals. Almond milk adds calcium and vitamin E, while chia seeds provide healthy fats and protein.

Cooking Time: This recipe takes about 10 minutes to prepare, plus overnight refrigeration.

Macrobiotic Cornbread

Ingredients:

✓ 2 ½ cups organic medium grind cornmeal

✓ 1 ½ cups unbleached organic white flour

✓ ¼ cup coconut oil

✓ ¼ cup maple syrup

✓ 2 cups non-dairy milk

✓ 2 teaspoons apple cider vinegar

✓ 2 teaspoons baking powder

✓ ½ teaspoon sea salt

Preparation:

1. Preheat oven to 375°F.

2. Coconut oil should be used to grease a 9-inch square baking dish.

3. In a large mixing bowl, whisk together cornmeal, flour, baking powder, and sea salt.

4. In a separate bowl, whisk together non-dairy milk, apple cider vinegar, coconut oil, and maple syrup.

5. Add the wet ingredients to the dry ingredients and stir until everything is well combined.

6. Smooth the top of the batter in the prepared baking dish.

7. A toothpick inserted in the center should come out clean after baking for 25 to 30 minutes, or until the cake is golden brown.

8. Allow a few minutes to cool before slicing it, then serve.

Nutritional Value: This dish is abundant in fiber, vitamins, and minerals. Cornmeal is a good source of complex carbohydrates and fiber, while coconut oil provides healthy fats. Non-dairy milk adds calcium and vitamin E, while maple syrup adds natural sweetness.

Cooking Time: This recipe takes about 40-45 minutes to prepare.

Bacon Roasted Potatoes

Ingredients:

✓ 6 large potatoes, unpeeled and cut into medium-sized cubes

✓ 6 slices of bacon, cooked and crumbled, reserving half of the bacon fat

✓ 1 onion, chopped

✓ 2 cloves garlic, minced

✓ 2 tablespoon of olive oil

✓ ½ teaspoon of sea salt

✓ ¼ teaspoon of black pepper

✓ ¼ teaspoon of dried thyme

✓ ¼ teaspoon of dried rosemary

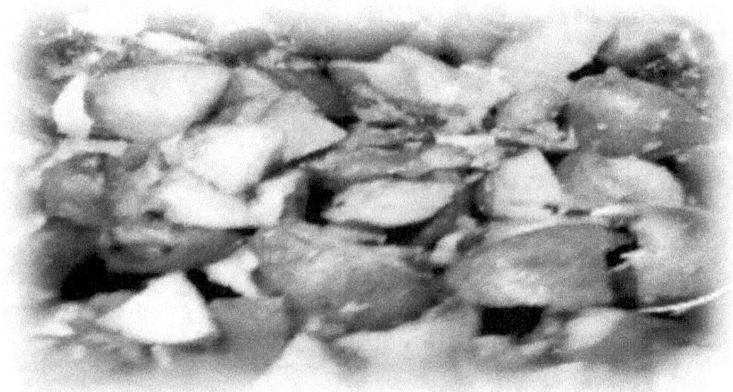

Preparation:

1. Preheat oven to 375°F.

2. In a large mixing bowl, combine potatoes, bacon, onion, garlic, olive oil, sea salt, black pepper, thyme, and rosemary.

3. Toss until everything is well coated.

4. On a baking sheet, apply the ingredients in a single layer.

5. Roast for 30-35 minutes, stirring occasionally, until the potatoes are golden brown and crispy.

6. Allow the dish to cool for a few minutes before serving.

Nutritional Value: This recipe is high in fiber, vitamins, and minerals. Potatoes are a good source of complex carbohydrates and fiber, while bacon provides protein and healthy fats. Olive oil offers antioxidants and healthy fats.

Cooking Time: This recipe takes about 45-50 minutes to prepare.

Carrot Hummus

Ingredients:

✓ 2 carrots, sliced and cooked till soft

✓ 2 cups cooked chickpeas

✓ ½ cup of chickpea water or spring water

✓ ¼ cup of tahini

✓ ¼ cup of fresh lemon juice

✓ 2 cloves garlic, minced

✓ ¼ teaspoon of sea salt

✓ ¼ teaspoon of black pepper

✓ ¼ teaspoon of cumin

✓ ¼ cup of olive oil

Preparation:

1. In a food processor, combine the steamed carrots, cooked chickpeas, chickpea water or spring water, tahini, fresh lemon juice, minced garlic, sea salt, black pepper, and cumin.

2. Pulse until smooth.

3. With the food processor running, slowly drizzle in the olive oil until the hummus is creamy and smooth.

4. You can either serve it right away or store it in the refrigerator for up to five days in an airtight container.

Nutritional Value: This recipe is high in fiber, vitamins, and minerals. Carrots are a good source of beta-carotene and other vitamins, while chickpeas provide protein and minerals. Tahini adds healthy fats and flavor, while garlic and cumin provide antioxidants and flavor.

Cooking Time: This recipe takes about 20-25 minutes to prepare, including the time to steam the carrots and cook the chickpeas.

Corn & Tofu Scramble

Ingredients:

✓ 3 onions, chopped

✓ 1 block tofu

✓ 2 cups sweetcorn, cooked

✓ 1 tablespoon sesame oil

✓ 3 tablespoons white miso

✓ 1 juice of one lemon

✓ 1 tablespoon olive oil

✓ ½ teaspoon herb salt

✓ 3 tablespoons water

✓ 1 handful parsley

Preparation:

1. Cook the onions in sesame oil for 5 minutes.

2. Stir in half cup of water, turn down the heat, and allow to cook for 1 hour so this is amazingly sweet and satisfying.

3. Add the herb salt, mix well, and sauté for a few more minutes stirring regularly.

4. Drain and scramble the tofu with your hands.

5. Mix in the sweet corn and tofu.

6. Mix the white miso, lemon juice, olive oil, and water.

7. Sprinkle over and mix into the tofu, onion, and corn mixture.

8. Serve with some freshly chopped parsley.

Nutritional Value: This recipe is high in protein, fiber, vitamins, and minerals. Tofu is a good source of protein and minerals, while sweet corn provides fiber and vitamins. Onions add flavor and antioxidants, while parsley provides vitamins and minerals.

Cooking Time: This recipe takes about 1 hour and 15 minutes to prepare, including the time to cook the onions.

Millet Chickpea Chard Carrot Breakfast Bake

Ingredients:

✓ ¼ cup uncooked millet (or ¾ cup cooked millet)

✓ 1 tablespoon flaxmeal

✓ ¼ cup chickpeas, cooked

✓ ¼ cup chard, chopped

✓ ¼ cup carrots, grated

✓ ¼ cup onion, chopped

✓ ¼ cup unsweetened almond milk

✓ ¼ teaspoon sea salt

✓ ¼ teaspoon black pepper

✓ ¼ teaspoon dried thyme

✓ ¼ teaspoon dried rosemary

Preparation:

1. Preheat oven to 375°F.

2. In a medium mixing bowl, combine millet, flaxmeal, chickpeas, chard, carrots, onion, almond milk, sea salt, black pepper, thyme, and rosemary.

3. Stir until everything is well combined.

4. Transfer the mixture to a prepared baking dish.

5. Bake for 25–30 minutes, or until golden and crispy brown.

6. Allow it cool for a few minutes before cutting it into slices, then serve.

Nutritional Value: This recipe is high in fiber, vitamins, and minerals. Millet is a good source of complex carbohydrates, protein, and fiber, while chickpeas provide protein and minerals. Chard and carrots add vitamins and minerals, while flaxmeal provides healthy fats and fiber.

Cooking Time: This recipe takes about 30-35 minutes to prepare.

Creamy Whole Rice Porridge

Ingredients:

✓ 1 cup short grain brown rice

✓ 3 cups water

✓ 1 pinch sea salt

✓ 1 cup organic apricots, washed off sulfur & left in water overnight

✓ ½ cup unsweetened almond milk

✓ ¼ cup maple syrup

✓ 1 teaspoon vanilla extract

✓ ¼ teaspoon cinnamon

Preparation:

1. Rinse brown rice and drain.

2. In a medium pot, bring water and sea salt to a boil.

3. Add brown rice and apricots, reduce heat to low, and simmer for 30-40 minutes, stirring occasionally.

4. Add almond milk, maple syrup, vanilla extract, and cinnamon to the pot. Stir until everything is combined.

5. Simmer on low for 5-10 minutes, until the porridge is creamy and thick.

6. Serve warm.

Nutritional Value: This recipe is high in fiber, vitamins, and minerals. Brown rice is a good source of complex carbohydrates and fiber, while apricots provide vitamins and minerals. Almond milk adds calcium and vitamin E, while maple syrup adds natural sweetness.

Cooking Time: This recipe takes about 50-60 minutes to prepare.

CHAPTER 3

Nourishing Lunches and Satisfying Dinners: Delicious and Balanced

Chunky Beetroot and Pumpkin Soup

Ingredients:

- ✓ 2 medium-sized beetroot bulbs, cut into small chunks
- ✓ 1 cup pumpkin, cut into small chunks
- ✓ 2 carrots, diced
- ✓ 1 onion, diced
- ✓ 1 tablespoon umeboshi puree
- ✓ 4 cups water
- ✓ ½ teaspoon sea salt
- ✓ ¼ teaspoon black pepper
- ✓ ¼ teaspoon dried thyme
- ✓ ¼ teaspoon dried rosemary

Preparation:

1. Bring the water and sea salt to a boil in a big saucepan.

2. Add beetroot, pumpkin, carrots, onion, umeboshi puree, black pepper, thyme, and rosemary to the pot.

3. Reduce heat to low and simmer for 30-40 minutes, until the vegetables are tender.

4. Remove from the fire and set aside for a few minutes to cool.

5. Using an immersion blender or a regular blender, blend the soup until smooth or until desired consistency is reached.

6. Serve warm.

Nutritional Value: This recipe is high in fiber, vitamins, and minerals. Beetroot is a good source of antioxidants and minerals, while pumpkin provides vitamins and fiber. Carrots add vitamins and minerals, while umeboshi puree provides a salty and sour flavor.

Cooking Time: This recipe takes about 45-50 minutes to prepare.

Brown Rice and Aduki Beans

Ingredients:

✓ 1 cup short grain brown rice

✓ ¼ cup aduki beans, soaked overnight

✓ 1 inch piece of kombu, rinsed

✓ 3 cups water

✓ ½ teaspoon sea salt

Preparation:

1. Rinse brown rice and aduki beans and drain.

2. In a medium pot, bring water and sea salt to a boil.

3. Add brown rice, aduki beans, and kombu to the pot, reduce heat to low, and simmer for 45-50 minutes, stirring occasionally.

4. Remove the kombu and discard.

5. Serve warm.

Nutritional Value: This recipe is high in fiber, vitamins, and minerals. Brown rice is a good source of complex carbohydrates and fiber, while aduki beans provide protein and minerals. Kombu adds iodine and other minerals.

Cooking Time: This recipe takes about 50-60 minutes to prepare.

Avocado Caesar Salad with Tempeh Croutons

Ingredients:

For the salad:

✓ 2 heads of romaine lettuce, chopped

✓ 1 avocado, sliced

✓ ¼ cup vegan parmesan cheese

✓ ¼ cup crispy tempeh croutons

For the tempeh croutons:

✓ 8 oz tempeh, cut into small cubes

✓ 2 tablespoon of tamari

✓ 1 tablespoon of fresh lemon juice

✓ 1 garlic clove, minced

✓ 1 teaspoon of maple syrup

✓ 1 tablespoon olive oil

For the dressing:

✓ 1 ripe avocado, pitted

✓ 2 garlic cloves, minced

✓ 2 tablespoon fresh lemon juice

✓ 1 teaspoon of dijon mustard

✓ ¼ cup water

✓ ¼ cup olive oil

✓ ¼ teaspoon of sea salt

✓ ¼ teaspoon of black pepper

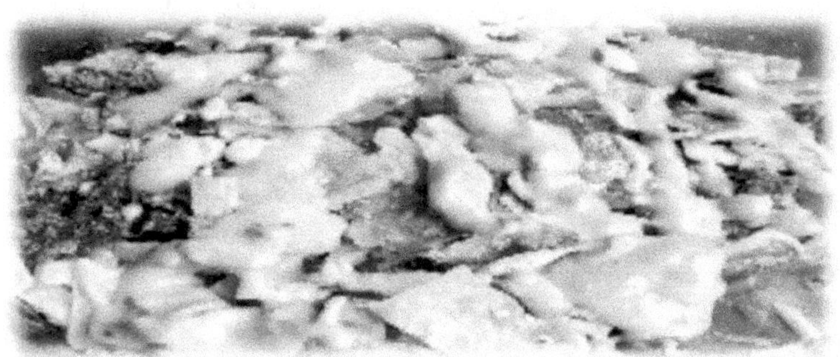

Preparation:

1. Preheat oven to 375°F.

2. In a mixing bowl, combine the cubed tempeh, tamari, fresh lemon juice, garlic, maple syrup, and olive oil. Cover and place in the refrigerator for at least 10 minutes to marinate.

3. Spread the tempeh cubes in a single layer on a baking sheet and bake for 20-25 minutes, until golden brown and crispy.

4. In a high-speed blender, combine the avocado, garlic, fresh lemon juice, dijon mustard, water, olive oil, sea salt, and black pepper. Blend until smooth and creamy.

5. In a large mixing bowl, combine the chopped romaine lettuce, sliced avocado, vegan parmesan cheese, and crispy tempeh croutons.

6. Drizzle the dressing over the salad and stir until evenly coated.

7. Serve immediately.

Nutritional Value: This recipe is high in fiber, vitamins, and minerals. Romaine lettuce is a good source of vitamins and minerals, while avocado provides healthy fats and fiber. Tempeh adds protein and minerals, while the dressing provides healthy fats and flavor.

Cooking Time: This recipe takes about 30-40 minutes to prepare, including the time to cook the tempeh.

Arugula Salad with Sautéed Mushrooms

Ingredients:

✓ 4 cups arugula

✓ 2 cups mushrooms, sliced

✓ ¼ cup onion, chopped

✓ 2 cloves garlic, minced

✓ 2 tablespoon of olive oil

✓ 1 tablespoon of tamari

✓ 1 tablespoon of fresh lemon juice

✓ ¼ teaspoon of sea salt

✓ ¼ teaspoon of black pepper

Preparation:

8. Warm the olive oil in a large pan over average heat.

9. Sauté the onion and garlic for 2-3 minutes, or until aromatic.

10. Add mushrooms and tamari and sauté for 5-7 minutes, until the mushrooms are tender and golden brown.

11. Remove from the fire and set aside for a few minutes to cool.

12. In a large mixing bowl, combine the arugula, sautéed mushrooms, fresh lemon juice, sea salt, and black pepper.

13. Toss until everything is well coated.

14. Serve immediately.

Nutritional Value: This recipe is high in fiber, vitamins, and minerals. Arugula is a good source of vitamins and minerals, while mushrooms provide protein and minerals. Olive oil provides healthful fats and antioxidants.

Cooking Time: This recipe takes about 15-20 minutes to prepare.

Macrobiotic Lunch Bowl

Ingredients:

✓ 1 cup cooked brown rice

✓ ½ cup cooked adzuki beans

✓ ½ cup sauerkraut

✓ ½ cup roasted sweet potato

✓ ½ cup steamed kale

✓ ¼ cup pickled ginger

✓ ¼ cup toasted sesame seeds

✓ 1 tablespoon of tamari

✓ 1 tablespoon of rice vinegar

✓ 1 tablespoon of olive oil

Preparation:

✓ In a large mixing bowl, combine the cooked brown rice, adzuki beans, sauerkraut, roasted sweet potato, and steamed kale.

✓ In a small mixing bowl, whisk together the tamari, rice vinegar, and olive oil.

✓ Drizzle the dressing over the bowl and toss until everything is well coated.

✓ Top with pickled ginger and toasted sesame seeds.

✓ Serve immediately.

Nutritional Value: This recipe is high in fiber, vitamins, and minerals. Brown rice is a good source of complex carbohydrates and fiber, while adzuki beans provide protein and minerals. Sauerkraut adds probiotics and vitamins, while sweet potato and kale provide vitamins and minerals.

Cooking Time: This recipe takes about 30-40 minutes to prepare, including the time to cook the brown rice and adzuki beans.

Brown Rice Green Bowl

Ingredients:

✓ ½ cup cooked brown rice

✓ 2 cups greens of your choice (baby kale, spinach, arugula, etc.)

✓ ½ cup broccoli florets

✓ ¼ cup tamari

✓ ¼ cup rice vinegar

✓ ¼ cup toasted sesame seeds

Preparation:

1. In a large mixing bowl, combine the cooked brown rice, greens, and broccoli florets.

2. In a small mixing bowl, whisk together the tamari, rice vinegar, and toasted sesame seeds.

3. Drizzle the dressing over the bowl and toss until everything is well coated.

4. Serve immediately.

Nutritional Value: This recipe is high in fiber, vitamins, and minerals. Brown rice is a good source of complex carbohydrates and fiber, while greens provide vitamins and minerals. Broccoli adds vitamins and minerals, while the dressing provides flavor and healthy fats.

Cooking Time: This recipe takes about 30-40 minutes to prepare, including the time to cook the brown rice.

Crispy Kale Salad

Ingredients:

✓ 1 huge bunch of kale, ripped off the stems and cut into pieces

✓ 2 teaspoons olive oil

✓ 2 teaspoons fresh apple cider

✓ ¼ teaspoon sea salt

✓ ¼ teaspoon black pepper

✓ ¼ teaspoon dried thyme

✓ ¼ teaspoon dried rosemary

✓ ¼ cup toasted sesame seeds

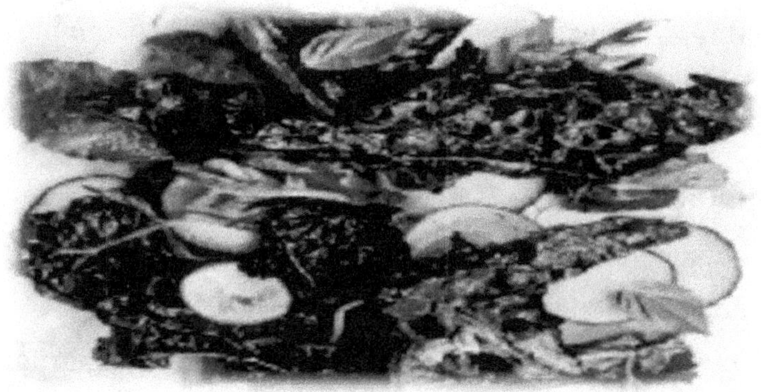

Preparation:

1. Preheat oven to 375°F.

2. In a large mixing bowl, combine the torn kale, olive oil, fresh apple cider, sea salt, black pepper, thyme, and rosemary.

3. Toss until everything is well coated.

4. On a baking sheet, arrange the kale in a single layer.

5. Bake for 10-15 minutes, until the kale is crispy and golden brown.

6. Remove from oven and set aside for a few minutes to cool.

7. Sprinkle with toasted sesame seeds.

8. Serve immediately.

Nutritional Value: This recipe is high in fiber, vitamins, and minerals. Kale is a good source of vitamins and minerals, while olive oil provides healthy fats and antioxidants. Sesame seeds add protein and minerals.

Cooking Time: This recipe takes about 20-25 minutes to prepare, including the time to bake the kale.

Brown Rice Buddha Bowl

Ingredients:

✓ ½ cup cooked brown rice

✓ ½ cup cooked adzuki beans

✓ 1 cup greens of your choice (baby kale, spinach, arugula, etc.)

✓ ½ cup roasted sweet potato

✓ ¼ cup pickled ginger

✓ ¼ cup toasted sesame seeds

✓ 1 tablespoon of tamari

✓ 1 tablespoon of rice vinegar

✓ 1 tablespoon of olive oil

Preparation:

1. In a large mixing bowl, combine the cooked brown rice, adzuki beans, greens, and roasted sweet potato.

2. In a small mixing bowl, whisk together the tamari, rice vinegar, and olive oil.

3. Drizzle the dressing over the bowl and toss until everything is well coated.

4. Top with pickled ginger and toasted sesame seeds.

5. Serve immediately.

Nutritional Value: This recipe is high in fiber, vitamins, and minerals. Brown rice is a good source of complex carbohydrates and fiber, while adzuki beans provide protein and minerals. Greens add vitamins and minerals, while sweet potato provides vitamins and fiber.

Cooking Time: This recipe takes about 30-40 minutes to prepare, including the time to cook the brown rice and adzuki beans.

Lentil and Vegetable Stew

Ingredients:

✓ 1 cup dried lentils, soaked overnight

✓ 1 onion, chopped

✓ 2 cloves garlic, minced

✓ 2 stalks celery, chopped

✓ 1 carrot, chopped

✓ ¼ swede, chopped

✓ 1 piece konbu

✓ 6 cherry tomatoes, halved

✓ 1 tablespoon olive oil

✓ 1 tablespoon tamari

✓ 1 tablespoon rice vinegar

✓ 1 tablespoon miso paste

✓ 4 cups water

✓ Salt and pepper to taste

Preparation:

1. In a large pot, sauté the onion, garlic, celery, carrot, and swede in olive oil until the vegetables are tender.

2. Add the soaked lentils, konbu, cherry tomatoes, tamari, rice vinegar, miso paste, and water.

3. Bring to a boil, then reduce heat and simmer for 30-40 minutes, or until the lentils are tender.

4. Season with salt and pepper to taste.

5. Serve hot.

Nutritional Value: This recipe is high in protein, fiber, vitamins, and minerals. Lentils are high in protein and fiber, while veggies are high in vitamins and minerals. Konbu adds iodine and other minerals, while miso paste provides probiotics and flavor.

Cooking Time: This recipe takes about 1 hour and 10 minutes to prepare, including the time to soak the lentils.

Seaweed Salad with Tofu

Ingredients:

✓ ½ cup dried wakame seaweed

✓ ½ block firm tofu, cubed

✓ ½ cup grated carrot

✓ ½ cup grated daikon radish

✓ ¼ cup chopped scallions

✓ 1 tablespoon sesame oil

✓ 1 tablespoon tamari

✓ 1 tablespoon rice vinegar

✓ 1 tablespoon toasted sesame seeds

Preparation:

1. Soak the dried wakame seaweed in cold water for 10-15 minutes, or until it has expanded and softened.

2. Drain and squeeze away any extra water from the seaweed.

3. In a large mixing bowl, combine the seaweed, cubed tofu, grated carrot, grated daikon radish, and chopped scallions.

4. In a small mixing bowl, whisk together the sesame oil, tamari, and rice vinegar.

5. Drizzle the dressing over the salad and toss to cover everything.

6. Sprinkle with toasted sesame seeds.

7. Serve immediately.

Nutritional Value: This recipe is high in protein, fiber, vitamins, and minerals. Seaweed is a good source of iodine and other minerals, while tofu provides protein and minerals. Carrot and daikon radish add vitamins and fiber, while scallions provide flavor and antioxidants.

Cooking Time: This recipe takes about 15-20 minutes to prepare, including the time to soak the seaweed.

Quinoa Stuffed Bell Peppers

Ingredients:

✓ 3-5 bell peppers, halved, seeds removed

✓ 2 cups quinoa, cooked

✓ 1/2 white onion, diced

✓ 1, (14.5 oz.) can diced tomatoes, drained

✓ 1 jalapeno, diced

✓ 1, (15 oz.) can low sodium black beans, rinsed and drained

✓ 1, (15 oz.) can of garbanzo beans, washed and rinsed

✓ 1, (15 oz.) can yellow corn, rinsed and drained

✓ 1 tablespoon chili powder

✓ ¼ teaspoon garlic powder

✓ ¼ teaspoon onion powder

✓ ¼ teaspoon red pepper chili flakes

✓ ¼ teaspoon dried oregano

✓ ½ teaspoon paprika

✓ Cheese (optional)

✓ Cilantro or hot sauce for garnish

Preparation:

1. Preheat the oven to 375°F.

2. In a large frying pan, heat the olive oil and sauté the onion for 2-3 minutes.

3. Cooked quinoa, black beans, garbanzo beans, corn, chopped tomatoes, jalapeo, and taco spice are all good additions.

4. Remove from heat after mixing everything together.

5. Fill the peppers all the way to the top with the quinoa filling.

6. Bake for 25-30 minutes, or until the peppers are soft, in a baking dish with the filled peppers.

7. Garnish with cheese (optional), cilantro, spicy sauce, or any other toppings you choose, and serve.

Nutritional Value: This dish is high in protein from quinoa, rich in antioxidants and vitamins from the vegetables, and offers a good balance of carbohydrates and fiber. The bell peppers provide an excellent source of Vitamin C, while quinoa offers a complete source of plant-based protein.

Preparation time: 15 minutes

Cooking time: 25-30 minutes

Buckwheat Noodles with Stir-Fried Veggies

Ingredients:

✓ 8 oz. buckwheat noodles

✓ 1/2 cup shiitake mushrooms, sliced

✓ 1/2 cup carrot, julienned

✓ 2 cloves garlic, minced

✓ 1 tablespoon of ginger, minced

✓ 1 cup napa cabbage, sliced

✓ ½ cup bell pepper, sliced

✓ 2 green onions, sliced

✓ 2 tablespoon of sesame oil

✓ 2 tablespoon of rice vinegar

✓ 1 tablespoon of maple syrup

✓ 2 tablespoons of tamari or low-sodium soy sauce

✓ 1 tablespoon of toasted sesame seeds

Preparation:

1. Cook the buckwheat noodles according to the package instructions until just al dente (7-8 minutes). Drain thoroughly.

2. Heat the sesame oil in a big frying pan or wok over average-high heat.

3. Add garlic and ginger and stir-fry for 30 seconds.

4. Add shiitake mushrooms, carrot, napa cabbage, bell pepper, and green onions and stir-fry for 2-3 minutes or until the vegetables are tender.

5. Add the cooked buckwheat noodles to the pan and stir-fry for another 1-2 minutes.

6. In a small bowl, whisk together rice vinegar, maple syrup, and low sodium soy sauce or tamari.

7. Pour the sauce over the noodles and vegetables and stir-fry for another 1-2 minutes.

8. Sprinkle with toasted sesame seeds and serve.

Nutritional Value: This dish is a balanced meal providing high-quality protein and fiber from buckwheat noodles, along with a variety of vitamins, minerals, and antioxidants from the mixed stir-fry vegetables. It's low in fat and high in nutrients.

Preparation time: 10 minutes

Cooking time: 10 minutes

Corn and Tofu Scramble

Ingredients:

✓ 3 onions, chopped

✓ 1 block tofu

✓ 2 cups sweetcorn, cooked

✓ 1 tablespoon sesame oil

✓ 3 tablespoons white miso

✓ 1 juice of one lemon

✓ 1 tablespoon olive oil

✓ ½ teaspoon herb salt

✓ 3 tablespoons water

✓ 1 handful parsley

Preparation:

1. Sauté the onions in sesame oil for 5 minutes, stir in half a cup of water, turn down the heat, and allow to cook for 1 hour so that it becomes sweet and satisfying.

2. Add the herb salt, mix well, and sauté for a few more minutes, stirring regularly.

3. Drain and scramble the tofu with your hands.

4. Mix in the sweetcorn and tofu.

5. Mix the white miso, lemon juice, olive oil, and water.

6. Sprinkle over and mix into the tofu, onion, and corn mixture.

7. Serve with some freshly chopped parsley.

Nutritional Value: Calories: 220, Fat: 11 g, Saturated Fat: 1.5 g, Carbs: 22 g, Fiber: 4 g, Protein: 12 g, Sugar: 7 g.

Preparation time: 10 minutes

Cooking time: 1 hour

Pasta and Pepper Salad

Ingredients:

✓ 2 cups wholegrain pasta, cooked

✓ 1 red pepper, cut into matchsticks

✓ 1 yellow pepper, cut into matchsticks

✓ ½ cup black olives

✓ 1 tablespoon sesame oil

✓ 1 tablespoon vegan pesto

✓ 1 tablespoon white miso

✓ 3 tablespoons water

Preparation:

1. Heat sesame oil in a pan and add peppers.

2. Sauté for 5 minutes, stirring frequently.

3. Add a generous pinch of salt and sauté for a further 10 minutes or until the peppers are soft.

4. Once the peppers are soft, turn off the heat and allow them to cool.

5. Stir in the cooked pasta and chopped olives.

6. Make the sauce by mixing pesto, white miso, and water.

7. Serve the pasta with the sauce on top.

Nutritional Value: Calories: 350, Fat: 12 g, Saturated Fat: 1.5 g, Carbs: 50 g, Fiber: 8 g, Protein: 12 g, Sugar: 3 g.

Preparation time: 10 minutes

Cooking time: 20 minutes

Vegan Avocado Caesar Salad with Tempeh Croutons

Ingredients:

✓ 2 heads of romaine lettuce, chopped

✓ 2 avocados, diced

✓ 1 tempeh packet, sliced into tiny cubes

✓ ½ baguette, cut into large chunks

✓ 4 cloves garlic, minced

✓ 1 tablespoon extra virgin olive oil

✓ ¼ cup cashews

✓ ⅛ cup pine nuts

✓ 1 garlic clove

✓ 2 teaspoons capers

✓ Juice of 1 lemon

✓ 1 teaspoon white miso

✓ ½ teaspoon dijon mustard

✓ ½ teaspoon agave nectar

✓ 2 tablespoons extra virgin olive oil

✓ ¼ cup water

✓ A few grinds of sea salt

Preparation:

1. Preheat the oven to 375°F.

2. Toss the tempeh cubes with tamari and bake for 15-20 minutes or until crispy.

3. Toss the bread chunks with minced garlic and olive oil and bake for 10-15 minutes or until crispy.

4. In a blender, combine cashews, pine nuts, garlic, capers, lemon juice, white miso, dijon mustard, agave nectar, extra virgin olive oil, water, and sea salt. Blend until smooth.

5. In a large bowl, toss the chopped romaine lettuce with the diced avocado and tempeh croutons.

6. Spread the dressing over the salad and mix to coat.

7. Serve with the garlic croutons on top.

Nutritional Value: Calories: 350, Fat: 22 g, Saturated Fat: 3 g, Carbs: 30 g, Fiber: 12 g, Protein: 14 g, Sugar: 4 g

Preparation time: 30-40 minutes

Cooking time: 25-35 minutes

Healthy Guacamole

Ingredients:

✓ 2 ripe avocados, peeled and pitted

✓ ¼ cup red onion, finely chopped

✓ ¼ cup fresh cilantro, chopped

✓ ½ lime, juiced

✓ ¼ teaspoon sea salt

✓ ¼ teaspoon black pepper

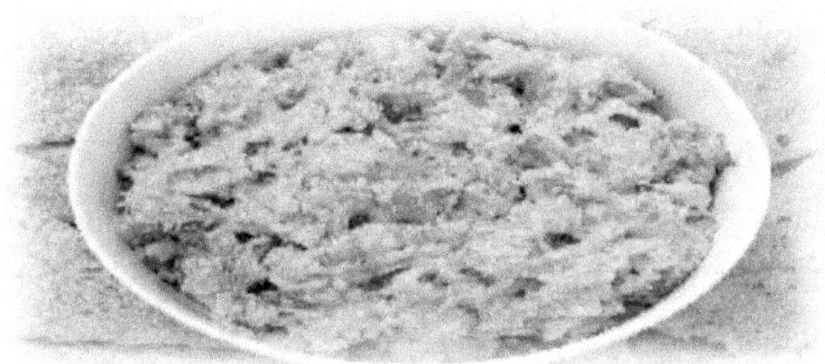

Preparation:

1. Mash the avocados using a fork or potato masher in a medium mixing basin.

2. Add the red onion, cilantro, lime juice, sea salt, and black pepper.

3. Mix well until all ingredients are combined.

4. Taste and adjust seasoning as needed.

5. Serve immediately with whole-grain crackers or sliced vegetables.

Nutritional Value: Calories: 160, Fat: 14 g, Saturated Fat: 2 g, Carbs: 9 g, Fiber: 7 g, Protein: 2 g, Sugar: 1 g

Preparation time: 10 minutes

Macrobiotic Brown Rice Stir-Fry with Veggies

Ingredients:

✓ 1 cup brown rice

✓ 2 cups water

✓ 1 tablespoon sesame oil

✓ 1 onion, sliced

✓ 2 cloves garlic, minced

✓ 1 carrot, sliced

✓ 1 cup broccoli florets

✓ 1 cup sliced mushrooms

✓ 1 tablespoon tamari

✓ 1 tablespoon rice vinegar

✓ 1 tablespoon maple syrup

✓ 1 tablespoon cornstarch

✓ ¼ cup of water

✓ 1 tablespoon sesame seeds

Preparation:

1. Bring to a boil, then lower to a low heat and continue to cook for 40-45 minutes, or until the rice is tender.

2. In a large pan over average-high heat, heat the sesame oil.

3. Cook the onion and garlic for 2-3 minutes.

4. Add carrot, broccoli, and mushrooms and sauté for another 5-7 minutes or until the vegetables are tender.

5. In a small bowl, whisk together tamari, rice vinegar, maple syrup, cornstarch, and 1/4 cup of water.

6. Stir-fry for another 1-2 minutes, or until the sauce thickens, over the veggies.

7. Serve over brown rice and sprinkled with sesame seeds.

Nutritional Value: Calories: 350, Fat: 10 g, Saturated Fat: 1.5 g, Carbs: 60 g, Fiber: 8 g, Protein: 10 g Sugar: 8 g.

Preparation time: 5 minutes

Cooking time: 50-55 minutes

Lentil Soup

Ingredients:

✓ 1 cup of dry lentils, soaked overnight in water

✓ 1 piece konbu

✓ 1 large onion, diced

✓ 2 cloves garlic, minced

✓ 1 carrot, sliced

✓ ¼ swede, diced

✓ 3 stalks celery, sliced

✓ 6 cherry tomatoes, halved

✓ Several slices fresh ginger

✓ ½ bunch parsley or coriander

✓ 1 tablespoon barley or rice miso

✓ 1 tablespoon olive oil

✓ Sea salt to taste

Preparation:

1. Discard the lentil's soaking water and cook them in plenty of fresh water until tender.

2. Dice the onion, garlic, carrot, swede, and celery and sauté in the olive oil for 10 minutes (starting with the onion) and then add these and the tomatoes to the lentils.

3. Simmer them together for another 10-15 minutes adding the miso and ginger slices.

4. Chop the parsley or coriander finely and add to the soup for the last few minutes of cooking.

5. Remove the konbu and ginger slices before serving and if necessary add some veggie stock to thin.

Nutritional Value: Calories: 200, Fat: 3 g, Saturated Fat: 0 g, Carbs: 32 g, Fiber: 16 g, Protein: 13 g, Sugar: 5 g.

Preparation time: 10 minutes

Cooking time: 30-40 minutes

Vegetable Stir-Fry with Soba Noodles

Ingredients:

✓ 8 oz soba noodles

✓ 2 tablespoon of sesame oil

✓ 2 cloves garlic, minced

✓ 1 onion, thinly sliced

✓ 1 cup broccoli florets

✓ 1 cup sliced mushrooms

✓ 1 carrot, sliced

✓ ½ cup snow peas

✓ ¼ cup tamari

✓ 1 tablespoon of rice vinegar

✓ 1 tablespoon of maple syrup

✓ 1 tablespoon of cornstarch

✓ ¼ cup water

✓ 1 tablespoon of sesame seeds

Preparation:

1. Cook soba noodles according to package instructions.

2. In a large pan over average-high heat, heat the sesame oil.

3. Cook the onion and garlic for 2-3 minutes.

4. Add broccoli, mushrooms, carrot, and snow peas and sauté for another 5-7 minutes or until the vegetables are tender.

5. In a small bowl, whisk together tamari, rice vinegar, maple syrup, cornstarch, and ¼ cup of water.

6. Stir-fry for another 1-2 minutes, or until the sauce thickens, over the veggies.

7. Sprinkle with sesame seeds and serve with soba noodles.

Nutritional Value: Calories: 350, Fat: 10 g, Saturated Fat: 1.5 g, Carbs: 60 g, Fiber: 8 g, Protein: 12 g, Sugar: 8 g.
Preparation time: 10 minutes

Cooking time: 20-25 minutes

Miso Glazed Tofu

Ingredients:

✓ 1 block extra-firm tofu

✓ 1 tablespoon miso paste

✓ 1 tablespoon rice-wine vinegar

✓ 2 tablespoons honey

✓ 1 tablespoon low-sodium soy sauce

✓ 1 tablespoon sesame oil

✓ 1 tablespoon cornstarch

✓ ¼ cup water

✓ 1 tablespoon sesame seeds

Preparation:

1. Preheat the oven to 375°F.

2. Cut the tofu into cubes and set them on a baking pan lined with parchment paper.

3. In a small bowl, whisk together miso paste, rice-wine vinegar, honey, soy sauce, and sesame oil.

4. Pour the mixture over the tofu and toss to coat.

5. Bake for 20-25 minutes or until the tofu is golden brown and crispy.

6. In a small mixing basin, combine cornstarch and water.

7. Heat sesame oil in a small saucepan over average heat.

8. Add the cornstarch mixture and whisk until the mixture thickens.

9. Drizzle the sauce over the tofu and sprinkle with sesame seeds.

Nutritional Value: Calories: 250, Fat: 12 g, Saturated Fat: 1.5 g, Carbs: 22 g, Fiber: 2 g, Protein: 16 g, Sugar: 14 g.

Preparation time: 10 minutes

Cooking time: 20-25 minutes

CHAPTER 4

Snacks, Desserts, and Treats for a Balanced Indulgence

Snacks

Brown Rice Cakes with Almond Butter

Ingredients:

✓ 1 brown rice cake

✓ 2 tablespoons almond butter (crunchy or creamy)

✓ ½ banana

✓ Cinnamon

Preparation:

1. Spread the almond butter over the rice cake.

2. Top with sliced bananas.

3. Sprinkle with cinnamon.

Nutritional Value: Calories: 200, Fat: 10 , Saturated Fat: 1 g, Carbs: 25 g, Fiber: 4 g, Protein: 6 g, Sugar: 10 g.

Preparation time: 5 minutes

Apple Slices with Tahini:

Ingredients:

✓ 1 apple, sliced

✓ 1 tablespoon tahini

✓ Cinnamon

Preparation:

1. Spread the tahini on the apple slices.

2. Sprinkle with cinnamon.

Nutritional Value: Calories: 120, Fat: 5 g, Saturated Fat: 1 g, Carbs: 20 g, Fiber: 4 g, Protein: 2 gSugar: 14 g

Preparation time: 5 minutes

Roasted Chickpeas

Ingredients:

✓ 1 can (440g | 15 oz) chickpeas, rinsed and drained - you can also use dry chickpeas. Soak them overnight.

✓ 2 teaspoons turmeric powder

✓ 1 teaspoon cumin powder

✓ 1 teaspoon coriander powder

✓ ½ teaspoon smoked paprika

✓ ½ teaspoon garlic powder

✓ ½ teaspoon onion powder

✓ ½ teaspoon sea salt

✓ 1 tablespoon olive oil

Preparation:

1. Preheat the oven to 400°F.

2. After rinsing and draining the chickpeas, blot them dry with a paper towel.

3. In a small bowl, mix together the turmeric powder, cumin powder, coriander powder, smoked paprika, garlic powder, onion powder, and sea salt.

4. In a large bowl, toss the chickpeas with the spice mixture and olive oil until they are evenly coated.

5. Spread the chickpeas in a single layer on a baking sheet lined with parchment paper.

6. Bake the chickpeas for 20-25 minutes, or until crispy and golden brown.

7. Allow to cool for a few minutes before serving after removing from the oven.

Nutritional Value: Calories: 161, Fat: 5 g, Saturated Fat: 0.5 g, Carbs: 23 g, Fiber: 6 g, Protein: 6 g.

Preparation time: 10 minutes

Cooking time: 20-25 minutes

Steamed Edamame

Ingredients:

✓ 1 lb. fresh or frozen edamame

✓ 2 teaspoons kosher salt

✓ Water

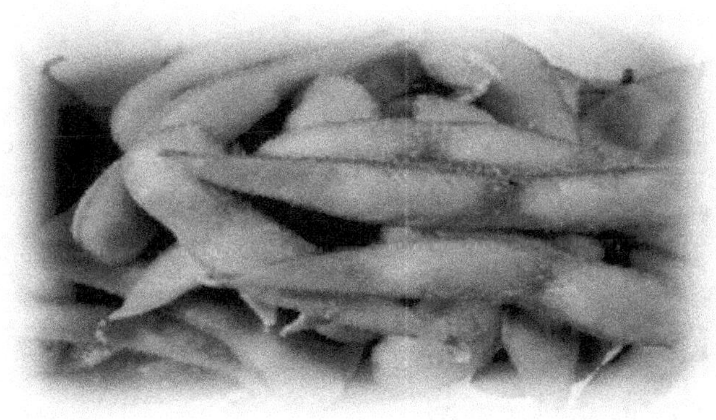

Preparation:

1. Pour water into a big pot to a depth of about ½".

2. Bring to a boil with 2 tablespoons kosher salt.

3. Place edamame in a steam basket and drop into pot.

4. Cover and steam for 8 to 10 minutes, or until the beans are completely soft. It may take longer if the food is frozen.

5. Drain the beans and place them in a large mixing dish.

6. Season with additional salt if desired.

Nutritional Value: Calories: 120, Fat: 5 g, Saturated Fat: 0.5 g, Carbs: 9 g, Fiber: 5 g, Protein: 11 g, Sugar: 2 g.
Preparation time: 5 minutes

Cooking time: 8-10 minutes

Nori Snacks

Ingredients:

✓ 4 sheets of nori seaweed

✓ 1 tablespoon sesame oil

✓ 1 tablespoon tamari

✓ 1 tablespoon rice vinegar

✓ 1 teaspoon honey

✓ ½ teaspoon grated ginger

✓ ½ teaspoon garlic powder

✓ ¼ teaspoon cayenne pepper

Preparation:

✓ Preheat the oven to 250°F.

✓ Cut the nori sheets into bite-sized pieces.

✓ In a small bowl, whisk together sesame oil, tamari, rice vinegar, honey, grated ginger, garlic powder, and cayenne pepper.

✓ Dip each piece of nori into the mixture, making sure it is fully coated.

✓ Place the nori pieces on a baking sheet lined with parchment paper.

✓ Bake for 10-15 minutes or until the nori is crispy.

✓ Allow to cool for a few minutes before serving after removing from the oven.

Nutritional Value: Calories: 40, Fat: 2 g, Saturated Fat: 0 g, Carbs: 4 g, Fiber: 1 g, Protein: 1 g, Sugar: 1 g.

Preparation time: 10 minutes

Cooking time: 10-15 minutes

Desserts

Baked Apples with Cinnamon

Ingredients:

✓ 4 medium apples

✓ 2 teaspoons cinnamon

✓ 1 tablespoon honey

✓ 1 tablespoon coconut oil

Preparation:

1. Preheat the oven to 375°F.

2. Cut off the top of each apple and scoop out the core and seeds.

3. In a small bowl, mix together cinnamon, honey, and coconut oil.

4. Stuff each apple with the mixture.

5. Place the apples in a baking dish and bake for 30-40 minutes or until the apples are tender.

6. Remove from the oven and set aside to cool for a few minutes before serving.

Nutritional Value: Calories: 120, Fat: 3 g, Saturated Fat: 2 g, Carbs: 25 g, Fiber: 5 g, Protein: 1 g, Sugar: 19 g.

Preparation time: 10 minutes

Cooking time: 30-40 minutes

Mochi with Red Bean Paste

Ingredients:

✓ 1 cup sweet rice flour

✓ 1/4 cup sugar

✓ 1/2 cup water

✓ 1/2 cup red bean paste

✓ Cornstarch

Preparation:

1. In a mixing bowl, whisk together sweet rice flour, sugar, and water until smooth.

2. Cover the bowl with plastic wrap and microwave for 2 minutes.

3. Remove from the microwave and stir the mixture with a spatula.

4. Cover the bowl again and microwave for another 1 minute.

5. Remove from the microwave and stir the mixture until it becomes a smooth dough.

6. Dust a work surface with cornstarch and roll out the dough to 1/4 inch thickness.

7. Cut the dough into small squares.

8. Place a small amount of red bean paste in the center of each square.

9. Pinch the edges of the dough together to seal the red bean paste inside.

10. To prevent sticking, roll each mochi ball with cornstarch.

Nutritional Value: Calories: 80, Carbs: 19 g, Fiber: 1 g, Protein: 1 g, Sugar: 8 g.

Preparation time: 10 minutes

Cooking time: 3 minutes

Date and Nut Balls

Ingredients:

✓ 1 cup pitted dates

✓ 1 cup mixed nuts (almonds, walnuts, pecans)

✓ ¼ teaspoon sea salt

✓ ½ teaspoon vanilla extract

✓ ¼ cup unsweetened shredded coconut

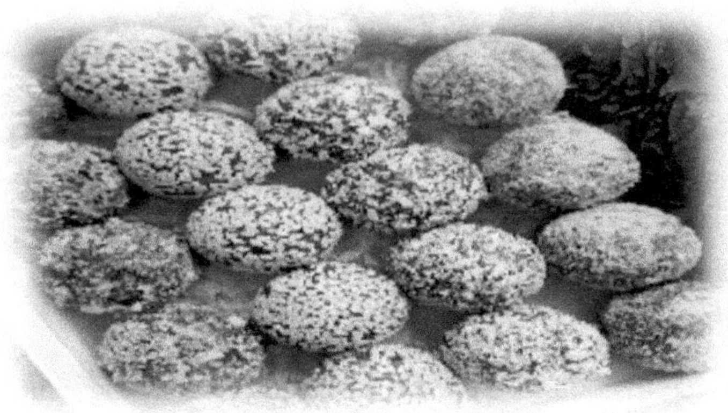

Preparation:

1. In a food processor, pulse the dates and mixed nuts until they are finely chopped.

2. Add the sea salt and vanilla extract and pulse until the mixture comes together.

3. Roll the mixture into small balls.

4. Roll the balls in the shredded coconut until they are coated.

5. Place the balls in the refrigerator for at least 30 minutes to firm up.

Nutritional Value: Calories: 100, Fat: 6 g, Saturated Fat: 1 g, Carbs: 11 g, Fiber: 2 g, Protein: 2 g, Sugar: 8 g.

Preparation time: 10 minutes

Cooling time: 30 minutes

Sweet Brown Rice Pudding

Ingredients:

- ✓ 1 cup sweet brown rice
- ✓ 3 cups water
- ✓ 1/4 cup maple syrup
- ✓ 1/2 teaspoon cinnamon
- ✓ 1/4 teaspoon nutmeg
- ✓ 1/4 teaspoon sea salt
- ✓ 1/2 cup raisins
- ✓ 1/2 cup chopped walnuts

Preparation:

- ✓ Rinse the sweet brown rice and drain.
- ✓ In a medium saucepan, combine the sweet brown rice and water.
- ✓ Bring to a boil, then lower to a low heat and cook for 45 minutes.
- ✓ Add the maple syrup, cinnamon, nutmeg, and sea salt to the rice.
- ✓ Stir in the raisins and chopped walnuts.
- ✓ Simmer for an additional 10-15 minutes or until the pudding is thick and creamy.
- ✓ Remove from the fire and set aside for a few minutes to cool before serving.

Nutritional Value: Calories: 200, Fat: 6 g, Saturated Fat: 0.5 g, Carbs: 36 g, Fiber: 2 g, Protein: 3 g, Sugar: 14 g.

Preparation time: 5 minutes

Cooking time: 1 hour

Poached Pears with Cardamom

Ingredients:

✓ 4-5 medium bosc pears

✓ ½ lemon

✓ 6 cups water

✓ ¼ cup brown sugar

✓ 2 cinnamon sticks

✓ 8 cardamom pods, cracked

✓ ¼ tsp ground ginger (or 1 tsp fresh ginger)

Preparation:

✓ Peel the pears, leaving the stems intact.

✓ Cut a thin slice off the bottom of each pear so that they can stand upright.

✓ Squeeze the lemon juice over the pears to prevent browning.

✓ In a large pot, combine water, brown sugar, cinnamon sticks, cardamom pods, and ginger.

✓ Bring the mixture to a boil, then reduce heat to low and add the pears.

✓ Simmer for 20-30 minutes or until the pears are tender.

✓ Remove the pears from the pot and let cool for a few minutes before serving.

Nutritional Value: Calories: 120, Carbs: 31 g, Fiber: 5 g, Protein: 1 g, Sugar: 22 g.

Preparation time: 10 minutes

Cooking time: 20-30 minutes

Treats

Homemade Popcorn with Nutritional Yeast

Ingredients:

✓ ¼ cup popcorn kernels

✓ 3 tablespoons nutritional yeast

✓ 2 tablespoons canola oil or avocado oil

✓ 1 teaspoon salt plus more as needed

Preparation:

1. Combine the nutritional yeast and salt in a large mixing bowl. To make seasoning easier, use a jar with a lid.

2. In a medium or big pot, heat the canola oil. Tilt the saucepan so that the oil coats the bottom.

3. Warm the saucepan over medium-high heat, then add three or four "test kernels," cover, and set aside.

4. Once the test kernels pop, add the remaining kernels and cover the pot.

5. Shake the pot occasionally to prevent burning.

6. Once the popping slows down, remove the pot from heat and let it sit for a few seconds.

7. Pour the popcorn into the container with the nutritional yeast and salt.

8. Cover the container and shake it until the popcorn is evenly coated.

Nutritional Value: Calories: 120, Fat: 6 g, Saturated Fat: 0.5 g, Carbs: 11 g, Fiber: 2 g, Protein: 5 g.

Preparation time: 5 minutes

Cooking time: 5-10 minutes

Dried Fruit and Nut Mix

Ingredients:

✓ 1 cup mixed nuts (almonds, walnuts, pecans)

✓ 1 cup mixed dried fruits (raisins, apricots, cranberries)

✓ ¼ teaspoon sea salt

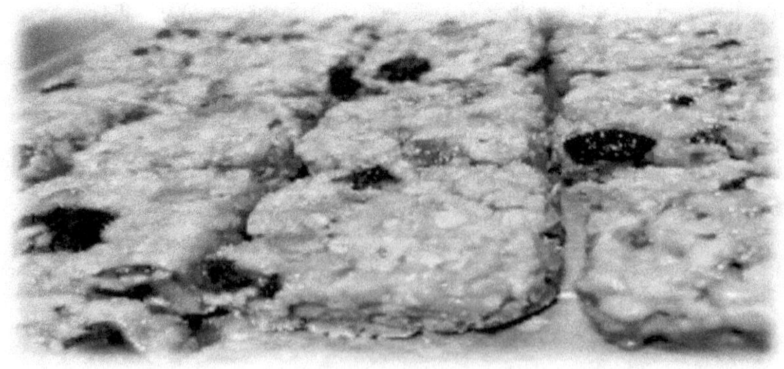

Preparation:

1. In a large bowl, mix together the mixed nuts, mixed dried fruits, and sea salt.

2. Store the mixture in an airtight container.

Nutritional Value: Calories: 150, Fat: 9 g, Saturated Fat: 1 g, Carbs: 17 g, Fiber: 2 g, Protein: 3 g, Sugar: 12 g.

Preparation time: 5 minutes

Matcha Green Tea Latte

Ingredients:

✓ 1 teaspoon matcha green tea powder

✓ 1 cup unsweetened almond milk

✓ 1 teaspoon honey or maple syrup (optional)

Preparation:

1. Warm the almond milk in a small saucepan over medium heat until it is warm but not boiling.

2. In a small bowl, whisk together the matcha green tea powder and a small amount of hot water to make a paste.

3. Add the matcha paste to the hot almond milk and whisk until it is fully combined.

4. To sweeten the latte, add honey or maple syrup to taste.

5. Pour the latte into a mug and serve immediately.

Nutritional Value: Calories: 60, Fat: 3 g, Carbs: 6 g, Fiber: 1 g, Protein: 2 g, Sugar: 4 g.

Preparation time: 5 minutes

Rice Crackers with Hummus

Ingredients:

✓ 4-6 brown rice crackers

✓ ½ cup cooked chickpeas

✓ 1 tablespoon tahini

✓ 1 tablespoon lemon juice

✓ 1 garlic clove, minced

✓ ¼ teaspoon sea salt

✓ ¼ teaspoon ground cumin

✓ ¼ teaspoon paprika

✓ 1 tablespoon olive oil

✓ Water, as needed

Preparation:

1. In a food processor, combine the chickpeas, tahini, lemon juice, garlic, sea salt, cumin, and paprika.

2. Pulse the ingredients until it is smooth and creamy.

3. With the food processor running, slowly drizzle in the olive oil until it is fully incorporated.

4. If the hummus is too thick, add water, 1 tablespoon at a time, until it reaches the desired consistency.

5. Spread the hummus onto the brown rice crackers and serve.

Nutritional Value: Calories: 120, Fat: 6 g, Saturated Fat: 1 g, Carbs: 13 g, Fiber: 3 g, Protein: 4 g, Sugar: 1 g.

Preparation time: 10 minutes

Vegetable Sushi Rolls

Ingredients:

✓ 2 Nori sheets, toasted

✓ 2 cups cooked brown rice

✓ 1 carrot, cut into matchsticks

✓ 1/2 cucumber, cut into matchsticks

✓ 12 tofu matchstick pieces

✓ 1 tablespoon mirin

Preparation:

1. On a sushi mat, place a nori sheet with the glossy side out and the lined side up.

2. Take a handful of brown rice and wet your hands (the water on your hands keeps the rice from sticking).

3. Line the nori sheet with brown rice, pressing it firmly into place.

4. Cover the entire nori sheet with brown rice, with the exception of 1.5cm at the farthest edge away from you, where you should leave a strip of nori to hold the sushi roll in place when rolling it.

5. When the nori sheet is mostly covered in brown rice, sprinkle with mirin. Take care not to overwet the rice.

6. Place the matchsticks horizontally along the nori sheet, 1 inch from the side closest to you. You should include a triumvirate of cucumber, carrot, and tofu.

7. Once the whole length of the nori sheet is covered in matchsticks, it's time to roll.

8. Cover the entire nori sheet with brown rice, with the exception of 1.5cm at the farthest edge away from you, where you should leave a strip of nori to hold the sushi roll in place when rolling it.

9. When the nori sheet is mostly covered in brown rice, sprinkle with mirin. Take care not to overwet the rice.

10.Place the matchsticks horizontally along the nori sheet, 1 inch from the side closest to you. You should include a triumvirate of cucumber, carrot, and tofu.

Nutritional Value: Calories: 250, Fat: 3 g, Carbs: 50 g, Fiber: 6 g, Protein: 8 g, Sugar: 3 g.

Preparation time: 15 minutes

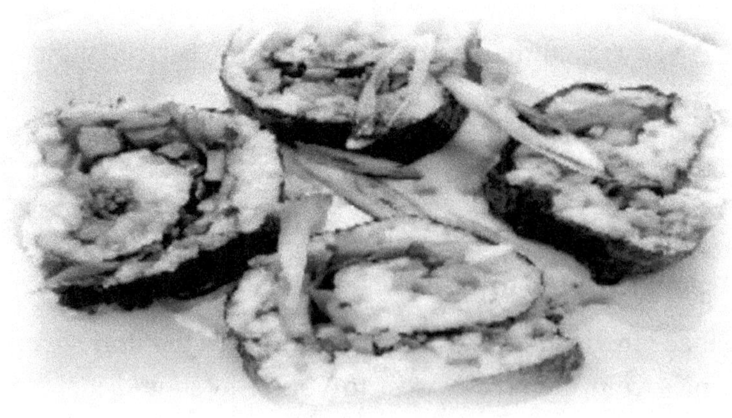

CHAPTER 5

Salads and Smoothies for a Finding Balance and Flavor

Salads

Quinoa and Vegetable Salad

Ingredients:

- ✓ 1 cup uncooked quinoa
- ✓ 2 cups water
- ✓ ½ teaspoon sea salt
- ✓ ½ cup chopped cucumber
- ✓ ½ cup chopped red bell pepper
- ✓ ½ cup chopped yellow bell pepper
- ✓ ½ cup chopped red onion
- ✓ ¼ cup chopped fresh parsley
- ✓ ¼ cup chopped fresh mint
- ✓ ¼ cup olive oil
- ✓ ¼ cup lemon juice
- ✓ 1 garlic clove, minced

Preparation:

1. In a fine mesh strainer, rinse and drain the quinoa.

2. In a medium saucepan, bring the water and sea salt to a boil.

3. Reduce to a low heat and add the quinoa.

4. Cook for 15-20 minutes, or until the water is absorbed and the quinoa is tender.

5. Remove the pan from the heat and put aside to cool.

6. Combine the chilled quinoa, cucumber, red bell pepper, yellow bell pepper, red onion, parsley, and mint in a large mixing basin.

7. In a small mixing dish, combine the olive oil, lemon juice, and garlic.

8. Pour the dressing over the quinoa mixture and toss to combine.

9. Serve chilled or at room temperature.

Nutritional Value: Calories: 200, Fat: 10 g, Saturated Fat: 1.5 g, Carbs: 24 g, Fiber: 4 g, Protein: 5 g, Sugar: 2 g.

Preparation time: 10 minutes

Cooking time: 20 minutes

Carrot and Daikon Salad

Ingredients:

✓ 2 medium carrots, peeled and grated

✓ 1 small daikon radish, peeled and grated

✓ 1 tablespoon toasted sesame oil

✓ 1 tablespoon rice vinegar

✓ 1 tablespoon tamari or soy sauce

✓ 1 tablespoon honey or maple syrup

✓ 1 garlic clove, minced

✓ ¼ teaspoon sea salt

✓ ¼ teaspoon black pepper

✓ 1 tablespoon sesame seeds, toasted

Preparation:

1. In a large bowl, combine the grated carrots and daikon.

2. In a small bowl, whisk together the sesame oil, rice vinegar, tamari or soy sauce, honey or maple syrup, garlic, sea salt, and black pepper.

3. Pour the dressing over the carrot and daikon mixture and toss to combine.

4. Sprinkle the toasted sesame seeds over the top of the salad.

5. Serve chilled or at room temperature.

Nutritional Value: Calories: 80, Fat: 4 g, Saturated Fat: 0.5 g, Carbs: 10 g, Fiber: 2 g, Protein: 2 g, Sugar: 6 g.

Preparation time: 10 minutes

Mixed Bean Sprout Salad

Ingredients:

✓ 2 cups mixed bean sprouts (mung bean, lentil, adzuki, etc.)

✓ ½ cup chopped cucumber

✓ ½ cup chopped red bell pepper

✓ ½ cup chopped yellow bell pepper

✓ ¼ cup chopped red onion

✓ ¼ cup chopped fresh cilantro

✓ ¼ cup chopped fresh mint

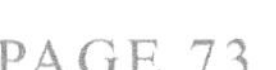

✓ 1 tablespoon toasted sesame oil

✓ 1 tablespoon rice vinegar

✓ 1 tablespoon tamari or soy sauce

✓ 1 garlic clove, minced

✓ ¼ teaspoon sea salt

✓ ¼ teaspoon black pepper

✓ 1 tablespoon sesame seeds, toasted

Preparation:

1. In a large bowl, combine the mixed bean sprouts, cucumber, red bell pepper, yellow bell pepper, red onion, cilantro, and mint.

2. In a small bowl, whisk together the sesame oil, rice vinegar, tamari or soy sauce, garlic, sea salt, and black pepper.

3. Pour the dressing over the mixed bean sprout mixture and toss to combine.

4. Sprinkle the toasted sesame seeds over the top of the salad.

5. Serve chilled or at room temperature.

Nutritional Value: Calories: 80, Fat: 4 g, Saturated Fat: 0.5 g, Carbs: 10 g, Fiber: 2 g, Protein: 4 g, Sugar: 3 g.

Preparation time: 10 minutes

Seaweed Salad with Miso Dressing:

Ingredients:

✓ ½ oz dried seaweed salad mix (approximately 1 handful)

✓ 1 tablespoon miso (koji miso or awase miso)

✓ 1 tablespoon soy sauce

✓ 1 tablespoon rice vinegar (unseasoned)

✓ 1 teaspoon roasted sesame oil

✓ 1 teaspoon mirin

✓ 1 garlic clove, minced

✓ ¼ teaspoon sea salt

✓ ¼ teaspoon black pepper

✓ ½ cup cherry tomatoes, halved

✓ 2 cups green leaf lettuce, chopped

Preparation:

1. Soak the dried seaweed salad mix in cold water for a few minutes to soften and then drain well.

2. In a small bowl, whisk together the miso, soy sauce, rice vinegar, roasted sesame oil, mirin, garlic, sea salt, and black pepper to make the dressing.

3. In a large bowl, combine the seaweed salad mix, cherry tomatoes, and green leaf lettuce.

4. Drizzle the miso dressing over the salad and toss to combine.

5. Serve chilled.

Nutritional Value: Calories: 70, Fat: 2 g, Carbs: 10 g, Fiber: 2 g, Protein: 4 g, Sugar: 3 g.

Preparation time: 10 minutes

Cucumber Wakame Salad

Ingredients:

✓ 20 grams of wakame sea vegetable

✓ 1 cucumber

✓ ½ teaspoon sea salt

✓ Zest and juice of half a lemon

✓ 1 tablespoon brown rice vinegar

Preparation:

1. Soak the wakame sea vegetable in cold water for a few minutes to soften and then drain well.

2. Cut the cucumber in half lengthwise and use a spoon to remove the seeds.

3. Slice the cucumber into thin half-moon shapes.

4. In a large bowl, combine the wakame sea vegetable and sliced cucumber.

5. In a small bowl, whisk together the sea salt, lemon zest, lemon juice, and brown rice vinegar.

6. Pour the dressing over the cucumber and wakame mixture and toss to combine.

7. Serve chilled.

Nutritional Value: Calories: 30, Carbs: 7 g, Fiber: 1 g, Protein: 1 g, Sugar: 2 g.

Preparation time: 10 minutes

Smoothies

Creamy Avocado Smoothie

Ingredients:

- ✓ 1 ripe avocado
- ✓ 1 banana
- ✓ ½ cup unsweetened almond milk
- ✓ ½ cup ice
- ✓ 1 tablespoon honey (optional)

Preparation:

1. Remove the pit from the avocado and scoop out the flesh.
2. Peel and chop the banana.
3. In a blender, combine the avocado, banana, unsweetened almond milk, and ice.
4. Blend until smooth and creamy.
5. If desired, sweeten the smoothie with honey.
6. Pour the smoothie halfway into a glass and serve.

Nutritional Value: Calories: 250, Fat: 15 g, Saturated Fat: 2 g, Carbs: 28 g, Fiber: 9 g, Protein: 4 g, Sugar: 14 g.

Preparation time: 5 minutes

Berry Blast Smoothie

Ingredients:

- ✓ 1 cup frozen mixed berries (raspberry, blueberry, strawberry mix)

✓ ½ cup unsweetened almond milk

✓ ½ cup ice

✓ 1 tablespoon honey (optional)

Preparation:

1. In a blender, combine the frozen mixed berries, unsweetened almond milk, and ice.

2. Blend until smooth and creamy.

3. If desired, sweeten the smoothie with honey.

4. Pour the smoothie halfway into a glass and serve.

Nutritional Value: Calories: 70, Fat: 2 g, Carbs: 14 g, Fiber: 4 g, Protein: 1 g, Sugar: 8 g.

Preparation time: 5 minutes

Green Smoothie

Ingredients

✓ 1 banana

✓ ½ cup unsweetened almond milk

✓ ½ cup frozen spinach

✓ ½ cup frozen kale

✓ ½ cup frozen pineapple

✓ 1 tablespoon honey (optional)

Preparation:

1. Peel and chop the banana.

2. In a blender, combine the banana, unsweetened almond milk, frozen spinach, frozen kale, and frozen pineapple.

3. Blend until smooth and creamy.

4. If desired, sweeten the smoothie with honey.

5. Pour the smoothie halfway into a glass and serve.

Nutritional Value: Calories: 120, Fat: 2 g, Carbs: 27 g, Fiber: 4 g, Protein: 3 g, Sugar: 15 g.

Preparation time: 5 minutes

Tropical Mango Smoothie

Ingredients:

✓ 1 banana

✓ ½ cup orange juice

✓ ½ cup frozen pineapple

✓ ¼ cup plain Greek yogurt

✓ ½ fresh mango

✓ 1 teaspoon honey (optional)

Preparation:

1. Peel and chop the banana and mango.

2. In a blender, combine the banana, orange juice, frozen pineapple, Greek yogurt, and fresh mango.

3. Blend until smooth and creamy.

4. If desired, sweeten the smoothie with honey.

5. Pour the smoothie halfway into a glass and serve.

Nutritional Value: Calories: 200, Fat: 1 g, Carbs: 47 g,

Fiber: 4 g, Protein: 5 g, Sugar: 33 g.

Preparation time: 5 minutes

Carrot-Orange-Ginger Smoothie

Ingredients:

✓ 1 small orange (140g)

✓ 1 medium carrot (60g)

✓ 1 slice fresh ginger, peeled (3-4g)

✓ ½ teaspoon turmeric powder

✓ ¼ teaspoon black pepper

✓ ½ cup unsweetened almond milk

✓ ½ cup ice

✓ 1 tablespoon honey (optional)

Preparation:

1. Peel the orange and chop it into small pieces.

2. Wash the carrot well and chop it into small pieces.

3. In a blender, combine the orange, carrot, fresh ginger, turmeric powder, black pepper, unsweetened almond milk, and ice.

4. Blend until smooth and creamy.

5. If desired, sweeten the smoothie with honey.

6. Pour the smoothie halfway into a glass and serve.

Nutritional Value: Calories: 70, Fat: 2 g, Carbs: 14 g, Fiber: 3 g, Protein: 1 g, Sugar: 9 g.

Preparation time: 5 minutes

CHAPTER 6

14 DAY MEAL PLANS

Below are 14-day macrobiotic meal plan that incorporates a variety of delicious and nutritious recipes:

Day 1

✓ **Breakfast:** Mediterranean Scrambled Tofu

✓ **Lunch:** Quinoa Stuffed Bell Peppers

✓ **Dinner:** Chunky Beetroot and Pumpkin Soup

✓ **Snack:** Brown Rice Cakes with Almond Butter

Day 2

✓ **Breakfast:** Buckwheat Pancakes with Fresh Fruit

✓ **Lunch:** Brown Rice Sushi Rolls

✓ **Dinner:** Lentil and Vegetable Curry

✓ **Snack:** Steamed Edamame

Day 3

✓ **Breakfast:** Miso Soup with Tofu and Wakame

✓ **Lunch:** Seaweed Salad with Tofu

✓ **Dinner:** Stir-Fried Brown Rice with Tofu

✓ **Snack:** Baked Apples with Cinnamon

Day 4

✓ **Breakfast:** Green Smoothie (Kale, Apple, Banana, Ginger)

✓ **Lunch:** Nori Rolls with Brown Rice and Veggies

✓ **Dinner:** Barley and Mushroom Risotto

✓ **Snack:** Roasted Chickpeas

Day 5

✓ **Breakfast:** Oatmeal with Berries and Almond Milk

✓ **Lunch:** Mediterranean Quinoa Salad

✓ **Dinner:** Steamed Edamame

✓ **Snack:** Date and Nut Balls

Day 6

✓ **Breakfast:** Sweet Brown Rice Pudding

✓ **Lunch:** Seitan Stir-Fry with Bok Choy

✓ **Dinner:** Quinoa Stuffed Portobello Mushrooms

✓ **Snack:** Carrot and Daikon Salad

Day 7

✓ **Breakfast:** Creamy Avocado Smoothie

✓ **Lunch:** Cucumber Wakame Salad

✓ **Dinner:** Lentil and Vegetable Stew

✓ **Snack:** Rice Crackers with Hummus

Day 8

✓ **Breakfast:** Buckwheat Noodles with Stir-Fried Veggies

✓ **Lunch:** Mixed Bean Sprout Salad

✓ **Dinner:** Tofu and Vegetable Lettuce Wraps

✓ **Snack:** Vegetable Sushi Rolls

Day 9

✓ **Breakfast:** Millet and Vegetable Stir-Fry

✓ **Lunch:** Brown Rice Cakes with Almond Butter

✓ **Dinner:** Quinoa Stuffed Bell Peppers

✓ **Snack:** Steamed Edamame

Day 10

✓ **Breakfast:** Mediterranean Scrambled Tofu

✓ **Lunch:** Seaweed Salad with Miso Dressing

✓ **Dinner:** Chunky Beetroot and Pumpkin Soup

✓ **Snack:** Date and Nut Balls

Day 11

✓ **Breakfast:** Buckwheat Pancakes with Fresh Fruit

✓ **Lunch:** Nori Rolls with Brown Rice and Veggies

✓ **Dinner:** Lentil and Vegetable Curry

✓ **Snack:** Roasted Chickpeas

Day 12

✓ **Breakfast:** Miso Soup with Tofu and Wakame

✓ **Lunch:** Quinoa Stuffed Portobello Mushrooms

✓ **Dinner:** Barley and Mushroom Risotto

✓ **Snack:** Brown Rice Cakes with Almond Butter

Day 13

✓ **Breakfast:** Green Smoothie (Kale, Apple, Banana, Ginger)

✓ **Lunch:** Seitan Stir-Fry with Bok Choy

✓ **Dinner:** Tofu and Vegetable Lettuce Wraps

✓ **Snack:** Baked Apples with Cinnamon

Day 14

✓ **Breakfast:** Oatmeal with Berries and Almond Milk

✓ **Lunch:** Mediterranean Quinoa Salad

✓ **Dinner:** Lentil and Vegetable Stew

✓ **Snack:** Steamed Edamame

This 14-day meal plan seeks to provide a balanced, diverse, and nutritious diet based on Macrobiotic Diet principles. Individual dietary needs and preferences should be considered when adjusting portion sizes and ingredients.

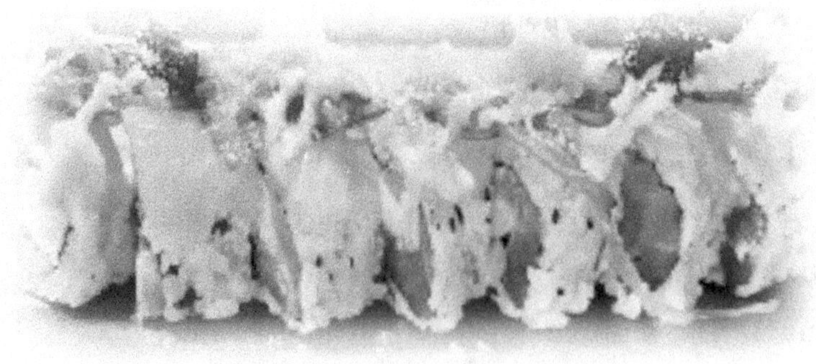

CONCLUSION

As we come to the end of our Macrobiotic Diet Cookbook, I'd like to take a moment to reflect on the incredible adventure you've been on. The recipes, which are based on millennia of knowledge, are more than simply meals; they represent your dedication to health, energy, and a harmonious relationship with the environment around you.

Your journey is more than simply what's on your plate; it's a profound connection to food's life-giving energy and the lively synergy between nature and human sustenance.

This cookbook has given you the tools you need to chart your own course toward long-term health and well-being. Accept balance, diversity, and awareness in all of your meals, and you'll experience a profound shift that goes beyond your body, including increased energy, clarity, and a deep sense of vitality.

Remember that information is your compass as you embark on your trip. Seek out resources, interact with like-minded people, and delve into the infinite knowledge of macrobiotic philosophy. This cookbook is only the beginning of a path to robust health and a lasting relationship to the profound wisdom of food.

Thank you for your interest in my macrobiotic diet cookbook. I am really grateful that you have decided to learn more about this way of life.

I understand that you have many cookbook options, so I am pleased that you chose mine. I poured my heart and soul into this book, and I hope it inspires you to prepare tasty and healthy meals that will benefit your entire health and well-being.

Macrobiotics has had a great influence on my life, and I am enthusiastic about educating people about the benefits of this way of living. Macrobiotics has taught me to listen to my body and eat what it needs when it requires it. It has also taught me how to cook in a way that protects nutrients while also enhancing flavor.

I hope this cookbook will assist you in reaping the same advantages from macrobiotics as I have. Please know that I am rooting for you while you create and enjoy the recipes in this book. I believe in you and in the ability of macrobiotics to change your life.

Here's a personal account of how macrobiotics have changed my life:

I was in my early twenties and was suffering from a variety of health conditions, including chronic exhaustion, stomach disorders, and skin problems. I did everything to improve myself, but nothing seemed to work.

Finally, I decided to give macrobiotics a go. I was apprehensive at first, but I needed relief so badly that I was prepared to give it a go.

I began to feel better after only a few weeks on the macrobiotic diet. My energy levels rose, my digestion improved, and my skin improved. My health improved so rapidly and profoundly that I was astounded.

I've been following the macrobiotic diet for a few years now, and my health has only improved. I am presently in better shape than I have ever been in my life.

I am quite appreciative of macrobiotics. It has restored my life.

I hope this cookbook will assist you in reaping the same advantages from macrobiotics as I have.

Thank you for your time in reading this cookbook.

If you have any concerns regarding macrobiotics or the recipes in this cookbook, please contact me at **loefflerlaura753@gmail.com.**

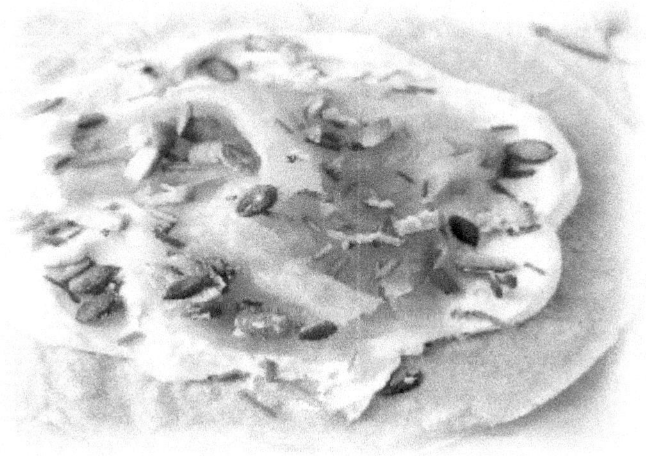

14 DAY MEAL PLANNER JOURNAL

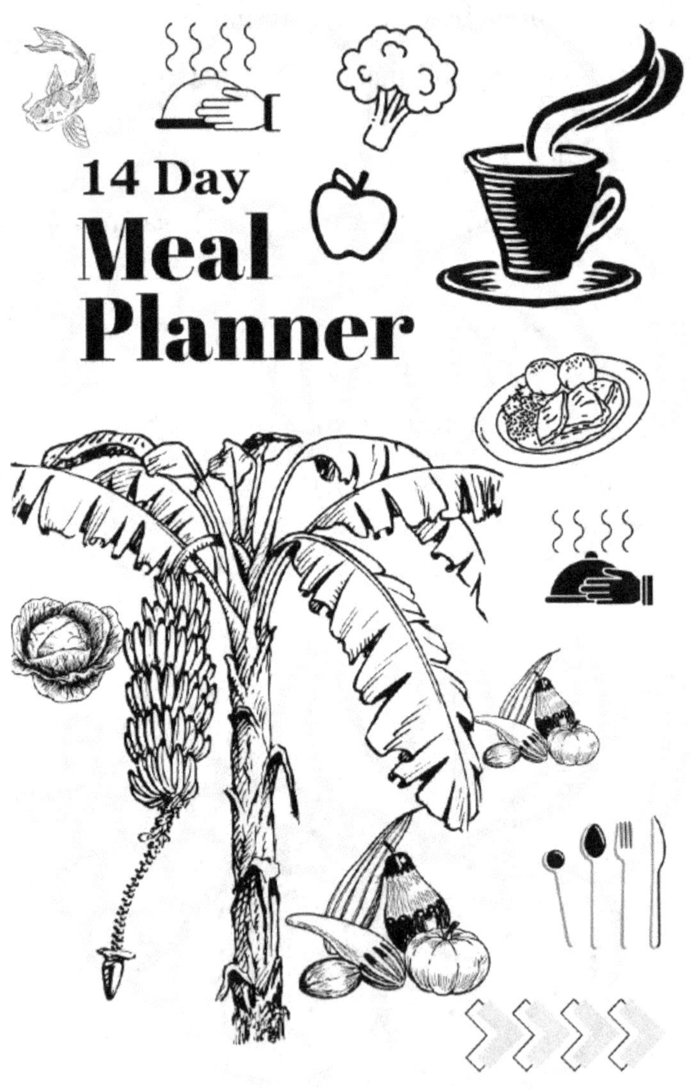

Menu List:

Breakfast:

Lunch:

Snacks:

Dinner:

Main Meal:

To Do List:

Shopping List:

TO BUY

SALAD

Note and Tips:

To-Do

Date/Day: Week:

Water: ▮ ▮ ▮

Menu List:

Breakfast:

Lunch:

Snacks:

Dinner:

Main Meal:

To Do List:

Shopping List:

☐ _______________

☐ _______________

☐ _______________

☐ _______________

☐ _______________

☐ _______________

TO BUY

SALAD

Note and Tips:

To-Do

Menu List:

Breakfast:

Lunch:

Snacks:

Dinner:

Main Meal:

To Do List:

Shopping List:

Note and Tips:

| Date/Day: | Week: | | Water: ■ ■ ■ |

Menu List:

Breakfast:

Lunch:

Snacks:

Dinner:

Main Meal:

To Do List:

____

____

____

____

____

Shopping List:

- ☐ ____________
- ☐ ____________
- ☐ ____________
- ☐ ____________
- ☐ ____________
- ☐ ____________

TO BUY

SALAD

Note and Tips:

To-Do

Date/Day: Week: Water:

Menu List:

Breakfast:

Lunch:

Snacks:

Dinner:

Main Meal:

To Do List:

Shopping List:

TO BUY

SALAD

Note and Tips:

To-Do

Date/Day: **Week:**   **Water:**

Menu List:

Breakfast:

Lunch:

Snacks:

Dinner:

Main Meal:

To Do List:

Shopping List:

Note and Tips:

Date/Day: Week:

Water:

Menu List:

Breakfast:

Lunch:

Snacks:

Dinner:

Main Meal:

To Do List:

Shopping List:

Note and Tips:

     MACROBIOTIC DIET COOKBOOK

Date/Day: **Week:**   **Water:**

Menu List:

Breakfast:

Lunch:

Snacks:

Dinner:

Main Meal:

To Do List:

Shopping List:

Note and Tips:

Water:

Menu List:

Breakfast:

Lunch:

Snacks:

Dinner:

Main Meal:

To Do List:

Shopping List:

TO BUY

Note and Tips:

To-Do

Menu List:

Breakfast:

Lunch:

Snacks:

Dinner:

Main Meal:

To Do List:

Shopping List:

TO BUY

SALAD

Note and Tips:

To-Do

Date/Day: **Week:**

Water: ☐ ☐ ☐

Menu List:

Breakfast:

Lunch:

Snacks:

Dinner:

Main Meal:

To Do List:

Shopping List:

☐ ______________
☐ ______________
☐ ______________
☐ ______________
☐ ______________
☐ ______________

TO BUY

~SALAD~

Note and Tips:

To-Do

Menu List:

Breakfast:

Lunch:

Snacks:

Dinner:

Main Meal:

To Do List:

Shopping List:

- ☐ __________
- ☐ __________
- ☐ __________
- ☐ __________
- ☐ __________
- ☐ __________

TO BUY

SALAD

Note and Tips:

To-Do

Menu List:

Breakfast:

Lunch:

Snacks:

Dinner:

Main Meal:

To Do List:

Shopping List:

Note and Tips:

Date/Day: **Week:**   **Water:**

Menu List:

Breakfast:

Lunch:

Snacks:

Dinner:

Main Meal:

To Do List:

Shopping List:

Note and Tips: